Copyright © 2023 by Lily J. Thompson (Author)

This book is protected by copyright law and is intended solely for personal use. Reproduction, distribution, or any other form of use requires the written permission of the author. The information presented in this book is for educational and entertainment purposes only, and while every effort has been made to ensure its accuracy and completeness, no guarantees are made. The author is not providing legal, financial, medical, or professional advice, and readers should consult with a licensed professional before implementing any of the techniques discussed in this book. The content in this book has been sourced from various reliable sources, but readers should exercise their own judgment when using this information. The author is not responsible for any losses, direct or indirect, that may occur from the use of this book, including but not limited to errors, omissions, or inaccuracies.

We hope this book has been informative and helpful on your journey to understanding and celebrating older adults. Thank you for your interest and support!

Title: Memory Matters-A Guide to Understanding and Supporting Older Adults with Dementia
Subtitle: Navigating Symptoms, Care, and Treatment

Series: Golden Living: A Guide to Aging Well Clues in the Community
By Lily J. Thompson

"The elders are the keepers of the flame, the guardians of the stories, and the carriers of the traditions."
Wendell Berry

"The elderly are treasures to society, carrying with them a wealth of knowledge and experience that cannot be replicated."
Hillary Clinton

"An elder is someone who has weathered the storms of life, and has emerged stronger, wiser, and more compassionate."
Dalai Lama

"The elders are like a lighthouse, guiding us through the storms and darkness of life, and showing us the way to safety."
Paulo Coelho

"Elders are the foundation of our communities, providing us with the stability, the wisdom, and the love that we need to thrive."
Desmond Tutu

"The elderly are not a burden on society, they are a gift. They have given us so much, and we must honor their contributions."
Queen Elizabeth II

"An elder is someone who has seen it all, done it all, and still has a sense of humor about it."
Betty White

Table of Contents

Introduction 7
   Importance of understanding dementia in older adults... 7
   Overview of the book's contents 10

Chapter 1: Understanding Dementia 13
   Definition and causes of dementia 13
   Types of dementia 15
   Early signs and symptoms 18
   Diagnosis and assessment 20

Chapter 2: Navigating Symptoms and Progression 23
   Stages of dementia and their characteristics 23
   Common symptoms and how to manage them 26
   Strategies for maintaining quality of life at each stage . 30
   Tips for caregivers and family members 34

Chapter 3: Approaches to Care and Treatment 38
   Holistic approaches to care, including non-pharmacological interventions 38
   Medications and their potential benefits and side effects 43
   Supportive services and resources for individuals with dementia and their caregivers 46
   Legal and financial planning considerations for dementia patients and their families 49

Chapter 4: Creating a Supportive Environment 52

Adapting the home environment to promote safety and independence 52
Creating a social support network for individuals with dementia and their caregivers 54
Incorporating meaningful activities into daily life 57
Addressing behavioral and psychological symptoms of dementia 60

Chapter 5: Addressing the Emotional Impact of Dementia 63

Coping with the emotional impact of a dementia diagnosis 63
Managing stress and burnout as a caregiver 66
Support and resources for family members and caregivers 69
Finding joy and connection in the midst of dementia 73

Chapter 6: Living with Dementia: Insights from Personal Experiences 76

Real-life stories of individuals and families living with dementia 76
Challenges faced and lessons learned 80
Coping strategies and tips for living well with dementia 83
Inspiring stories of resilience and hope 86

Conclusion 88

Recap of key takeaways from the book 88
Call to action for readers to engage with and support the elder population living with dementia in their communities...90
Final thoughts and encouragement for readers to navigate the complexities of dementia with empathy, understanding, and resilience...92

Key Terms and Definitions 96

Supporting Materials..99

Introduction
Importance of understanding dementia in older adults

As the population ages, the prevalence of dementia continues to increase. In fact, according to the World Health Organization (WHO), around 50 million people worldwide are living with dementia, and this number is expected to triple by 2050. Dementia is a syndrome that affects memory, thinking, behavior, and the ability to perform everyday activities. It can be caused by various factors, including Alzheimer's disease, vascular dementia, Lewy body dementia, and frontotemporal dementia.

Dementia not only affects the individuals living with it but also their families, caregivers, and communities. It can be a challenging and complex disease to manage, and it requires a multidisciplinary approach that involves healthcare professionals, social workers, and caregivers. Therefore, it's crucial to have a basic understanding of dementia, its symptoms, progression, and available treatment options.

Understanding dementia can help older adults and their families recognize the early signs and symptoms of the disease, seek early diagnosis and intervention, and plan for the future. Early diagnosis and intervention can help delay the progression of symptoms, improve the quality of life for individuals living with dementia, and reduce the burden on caregivers and families.

Moreover, understanding dementia can also help reduce stigma and misconceptions surrounding the disease. Dementia is often associated with aging, and many people believe that it's a normal part of the aging process. However, dementia is not a normal part of aging, and it's important to recognize that it's a disease that requires specialized care and support.

By understanding dementia, older adults and their families can also better navigate the healthcare system and access available resources and support services. These resources may include healthcare professionals specializing in dementia care, community-based services, and respite care for caregivers.

In summary, the importance of understanding dementia in older adults cannot be overstated. It's a complex and challenging disease that requires a multidisciplinary approach and specialized care. By recognizing the early signs and symptoms of dementia, seeking early diagnosis and intervention, and accessing available resources and support services, individuals living with dementia and their families can better manage the disease and improve their quality of life.

Overview of the book's contents

Memory Matters: A Guide to Understanding and Supporting Older Adults with Dementia is a comprehensive guide that provides readers with an in-depth understanding of dementia, its symptoms, care, and treatment. This book is intended for anyone who is interested in learning about dementia, including family members, caregivers, and healthcare professionals.

The book is divided into five chapters, each of which addresses a specific aspect of dementia care. Chapter 1, "Understanding Dementia," provides an overview of dementia, including its definition, causes, types, and early signs and symptoms. It also covers the diagnosis and assessment process.

Chapter 2, "Navigating Symptoms and Progression," focuses on the various stages of dementia and their characteristics, as well as common symptoms and how to manage them. The chapter also provides strategies for maintaining quality of life at each stage and tips for caregivers and family members.

Chapter 3, "Approaches to Care and Treatment," covers the holistic approaches to care, including non-pharmacological interventions, medications and their potential benefits and side effects, supportive services and resources for individuals with dementia and their caregivers, and legal and financial planning considerations for dementia patients and their families.

Chapter 4, "Creating a Supportive Environment," discusses how to adapt the home environment to promote safety and independence, create a social support network for individuals with dementia and their caregivers, and incorporate meaningful activities into daily life. The chapter also addresses behavioral and psychological symptoms of dementia.

Chapter 5, "Addressing the Emotional Impact of Dementia," provides guidance on coping with the emotional impact of a dementia diagnosis, managing stress and burnout as a caregiver, and finding support and resources for family members and caregivers. It also highlights ways to find joy and connection in the midst of dementia.

Each chapter includes practical advice, tips, and real-life examples to help readers better understand and navigate the complexities of dementia care. The book also includes a conclusion that summarizes the key takeaways and encourages readers to engage with and support the elder population living with dementia in their communities.

Overall, Memory Matters is an essential guide that empowers readers with the knowledge and skills needed to provide quality care and support to individuals with dementia and their families.

Chapter 1: Understanding Dementia
Definition and causes of dementia

Dementia is a term that refers to a group of progressive neurological disorders that affect memory, thinking, behavior, and daily activities. It is characterized by a decline in cognitive function beyond what is considered a normal part of aging, and it can have a significant impact on a person's quality of life.

The most common cause of dementia is Alzheimer's disease, which accounts for about 60-80% of cases. Other causes include vascular dementia, Lewy body dementia, frontotemporal dementia, and mixed dementia. In some cases, dementia may be caused by a combination of factors, including genetics, lifestyle, and environmental factors.

Alzheimer's disease is a neurodegenerative disorder that is characterized by the accumulation of two abnormal proteins in the brain: beta-amyloid and tau. These proteins form plaques and tangles, which interfere with the normal communication between brain cells and eventually lead to cell death. Vascular dementia, on the other hand, is caused by a reduction in blood flow to the brain, which can result from conditions such as stroke or high blood pressure.

Lewy body dementia is a type of dementia that is caused by the accumulation of abnormal proteins in the brain called Lewy bodies. These proteins are similar to those found in Parkinson's disease, and the symptoms of Lewy body dementia can include tremors, stiffness, and difficulty with movement, as well as cognitive and behavioral symptoms.

Frontotemporal dementia is a type of dementia that affects the frontal and temporal lobes of the brain, which are responsible for behavior, language, and executive functions. It can lead to changes in personality, language difficulties, and problems with social behavior and decision-making.

Mixed dementia is a combination of two or more types of dementia, often Alzheimer's disease and vascular dementia.

In summary, dementia is a complex and multifactorial disorder that can be caused by a variety of factors, including genetics, lifestyle, and environmental factors. Understanding the different types of dementia and their underlying causes is essential for effective diagnosis and treatment.

Types of dementia

Dementia is a broad term that encompasses various conditions characterized by cognitive decline and memory loss. Different types of dementia are associated with specific causes and patterns of symptoms. In this chapter, we will explore the various types of dementia and their unique features.

Alzheimer's Disease

Alzheimer's disease is the most common type of dementia, accounting for 60-80% of all dementia cases. It is a progressive disease that affects memory, thinking, and behavior. The exact cause of Alzheimer's is unknown, but it is believed to be linked to the accumulation of beta-amyloid plaques and tau protein tangles in the brain. Some of the key symptoms of Alzheimer's disease include memory loss, difficulty with language and communication, confusion, and changes in mood and behavior.

Vascular Dementia

Vascular dementia is the second most common type of dementia, accounting for about 10% of all cases. It is caused by reduced blood flow to the brain due to damage to the blood vessels. This damage can be caused by a stroke, atherosclerosis, or other cardiovascular conditions. Vascular dementia can cause a range of symptoms, including difficulty with organization and planning, memory problems, and changes in personality.

Lewy Body Dementia

Lewy body dementia is characterized by the accumulation of abnormal protein deposits called Lewy bodies in the brain. It is the third most common type of dementia and accounts for about 5-10% of all cases. Some of the key symptoms of Lewy body dementia include fluctuations in alertness and attention, visual hallucinations, and movement problems similar to those seen in Parkinson's disease.

Frontotemporal Dementia

Frontotemporal dementia is a group of disorders that affect the frontal and temporal lobes of the brain. These areas are responsible for personality, behavior, and language. Frontotemporal dementia is less common than Alzheimer's and vascular dementia, accounting for about 5% of all dementia cases. The symptoms of frontotemporal dementia depend on which part of the brain is affected, but can include changes in behavior, speech problems, and difficulty with movement.

Mixed Dementia

Mixed dementia is a combination of two or more types of dementia, often Alzheimer's disease and vascular dementia. It is estimated that about 10-20% of all dementia cases are mixed dementia. The symptoms of mixed dementia can vary depending on the types of dementia involved.

Other Types of Dementia

In addition to the four main types of dementia, there are several other types that are less common. These include Huntington's disease, Parkinson's disease dementia, and Creutzfeldt-Jakob disease. Each of these types of dementia has its own unique set of symptoms and causes.

Understanding the different types of dementia is important for both caregivers and individuals with dementia. It can help with early detection, diagnosis, and treatment, as well as provide insight into what to expect as the disease progresses. In the next section, we will discuss the early signs and symptoms of dementia.

Early signs and symptoms

Dementia is a progressive disease that affects the brain and cognitive function. The onset of symptoms can be gradual and may go unnoticed in its early stages. However, early detection and intervention can help slow down the progression of the disease and improve the quality of life for those affected. In this section, we will discuss the early signs and symptoms of dementia that individuals, caregivers, and healthcare providers should be aware of.

Memory Loss Memory loss is one of the most common early signs of dementia. Individuals may have difficulty remembering recent events or information, such as appointments, conversations, or activities they just did. They may also struggle with recalling names or faces of people they know well.

Difficulty with Language and Communication As dementia progresses, individuals may experience difficulty finding the right words, forming sentences, or following conversations. They may also struggle with reading and writing.

Confusion and Disorientation Individuals with dementia may become confused about time, place, and identity. They may forget where they are, how they got there, or where they are going. They may also have trouble recognizing familiar places, objects, or people.

Mood and Personality Changes Dementia can also cause mood swings, anxiety, depression, and irritability. Individuals may become withdrawn, lose interest in their hobbies, or have difficulty expressing emotions.

Impaired Judgement and Problem-Solving Skills As dementia progresses, individuals may have difficulty making decisions, solving problems, or handling money. They may also have poor judgement and may engage in risky behaviors.

It's important to note that these early signs and symptoms of dementia may not necessarily indicate the presence of the disease. Other factors, such as stress, anxiety, or depression, can also cause similar symptoms. However, if these symptoms persist or worsen over time, it's important to seek medical attention for a proper diagnosis and treatment.

Diagnosis and assessment

Diagnosis and assessment are critical aspects of understanding and managing dementia. Accurate diagnosis of dementia is crucial because it can affect the course of the disease, and early diagnosis can lead to better treatment outcomes. In this section, we will discuss the different methods used for diagnosing dementia and how assessments can help in the management of the disease.

Diagnostic Criteria Dementia diagnosis is typically based on a comprehensive medical evaluation, including medical history, physical and neurological examination, cognitive tests, and laboratory tests. The criteria for diagnosing dementia are established by organizations such as the American Psychiatric Association and the National Institute on Aging-Alzheimer's Association.

Medical History and Physical Examination A medical history can provide insight into the patient's symptoms and medical conditions, including risk factors for dementia. The physical examination is conducted to check for any underlying medical conditions that could be causing the symptoms.

Cognitive Tests Cognitive tests assess the individual's thinking, memory, and ability to solve problems. The tests may include the Mini-Mental State Examination (MMSE),

Montreal Cognitive Assessment (MoCA), and other tests that evaluate cognitive abilities.

Neurological Tests Neurological tests can help determine if there are any neurological conditions causing the symptoms. These tests may include a brain scan, such as magnetic resonance imaging (MRI) or computed tomography (CT), which can detect brain changes associated with dementia.

Assessing Disease Progression Assessing the progression of dementia is essential to ensure that patients receive the appropriate care and support. It can also help caregivers and family members anticipate changes in behavior and provide the necessary care. The following assessments are commonly used to evaluate the progression of dementia:

Global Deterioration Scale (GDS) The GDS is used to stage the progression of dementia based on cognitive and functional impairment. It ranges from Stage 1 (no cognitive decline) to Stage 7 (severe dementia).

Clinical Dementia Rating (CDR) The CDR is a tool used to assess the severity of dementia. It measures cognitive and functional impairment, and rates the severity of dementia on a scale of 0 to 3.

Functional Assessment Staging (FAST) FAST is used to assess functional impairment in dementia patients. It ranges from Stage 1 (normal functioning) to Stage 7 (total dependence).

In summary, diagnosing and assessing dementia is a complex process that requires a thorough medical evaluation. Early detection and diagnosis can improve the quality of life for individuals with dementia and their families. Careful monitoring of disease progression through assessments can help in providing appropriate care and support.

Chapter 2: Navigating Symptoms and Progression
Stages of dementia and their characteristics

Dementia is a progressive disease, meaning it worsens over time. The progression of the disease is typically divided into stages, although the exact duration and symptoms of each stage can vary from person to person. Understanding the stages of dementia can help caregivers and family members provide appropriate care and support, and can also help individuals with dementia maintain their quality of life as long as possible.

Mild Cognitive Impairment (MCI)

Mild Cognitive Impairment (MCI) is considered the earliest stage of dementia. It is characterized by memory problems, difficulty with language and communication, and changes in mood or behavior. However, individuals with MCI are still able to perform their activities of daily living, and the symptoms do not yet interfere significantly with their daily functioning. In some cases, MCI may not progress to dementia.

Early Stage Dementia

The early stage of dementia is marked by increasing memory loss and difficulty with communication. Individuals with early stage dementia may have difficulty remembering new information, completing tasks that require concentration or organization, or following conversations. They may also experience changes in personality or behavior, such as increased irritability or apathy. However, they are still able to perform many activities of daily living and may not require full-time care.

Middle Stage Dementia

In the middle stage of dementia, symptoms become more severe and the individual's ability to perform activities of daily living declines. Memory loss is more significant, and individuals may become disoriented or confused about time, place, and people. They may have difficulty with basic self-care tasks such as bathing and dressing, and may experience incontinence. Communication becomes more difficult, and individuals may have trouble finding the right words or understanding complex instructions. Behavioral changes such as agitation, aggression, or wandering may also occur.

Late Stage Dementia

In the late stage of dementia, individuals become completely dependent on caregivers for all their needs. They may be unable to walk or move independently, and may be bedridden. Communication is severely impaired, and individuals may be unable to speak or understand language. They may experience difficulty swallowing and may be at risk for infections and other health complications. In the final stages of the disease, the individual may become unresponsive and may require round-the-clock care.

It's important to note that the progression of dementia can be unpredictable, and not all individuals will experience all of these stages. Additionally, the duration of each stage can vary widely, with some individuals remaining in the early stage for several years and others progressing rapidly through the stages. However, understanding the general characteristics of each stage can help caregivers and family members provide appropriate care and support to individuals with dementia.

Common symptoms and how to manage them

Dementia is a complex disease that affects various cognitive, functional, and behavioral abilities. The symptoms of dementia can vary depending on the type and stage of the disease, and they often worsen as the disease progresses. Therefore, it is essential for caregivers and family members to understand the common symptoms of dementia and how to manage them effectively to ensure the safety, well-being, and quality of life of individuals with dementia. In this section, we will discuss the most common symptoms of dementia and the approaches to managing them.

Memory Impairment: Memory loss is one of the most common symptoms of dementia, particularly in the early stages of the disease. People with dementia may have difficulty remembering recent events, names, and faces, and may rely on notes or reminders to complete daily tasks. To manage memory impairment, caregivers can:

Use memory aids: Simple tools such as calendars, notes, or lists can help individuals with dementia remember important information and appointments.

Provide structure and routine: Establishing a consistent daily routine and structuring activities can help individuals with dementia feel more in control and reduce confusion.

Engage in reminiscence therapy: Encouraging individuals with dementia to recall positive memories from the past can help improve their mood and overall well-being.

Communication Difficulties: Dementia can affect the ability to communicate effectively, causing individuals to struggle with finding the right words, following conversations, or understanding nonverbal cues. To manage communication difficulties, caregivers can:

Use simple language: Speak in a clear and concise manner, using simple and familiar words and phrases.

Practice active listening: Pay attention to the individual's body language and tone of voice, and respond appropriately.

Use visual aids: Pictures, gestures, or other visual aids can help individuals with dementia better understand and remember information.

Behavioral and Psychological Symptoms: Dementia can also cause a range of behavioral and psychological symptoms, such as agitation, aggression, depression, or hallucinations. These symptoms can be challenging to manage and may require medication or other interventions. To manage these symptoms, caregivers can:

Identify triggers: Understanding the underlying causes of behavioral and psychological symptoms can help prevent or minimize their occurrence.

Use non-pharmacological interventions: Strategies such as music therapy, art therapy, or sensory stimulation can help reduce agitation and improve mood.

Consider medication: In some cases, medication may be necessary to manage severe symptoms of dementia, but it should be used with caution and under medical supervision.

Physical Changes: Dementia can also lead to physical changes, such as difficulty walking, balance problems, or incontinence. These changes can affect the individual's mobility and increase the risk of falls or other accidents. To manage physical changes, caregivers can:

Ensure a safe environment: Removing obstacles, installing grab bars or handrails, and ensuring adequate lighting can help reduce the risk of falls.

Provide physical therapy: Exercises and physical therapy can help maintain mobility and prevent further decline.

Use assistive devices: Devices such as walkers, canes, or wheelchairs can help individuals with dementia remain independent and safe.

In conclusion, managing the common symptoms of dementia requires a multifaceted approach that addresses the individual's physical, cognitive, and emotional needs. Caregivers and family members can use a range of strategies, including memory aids, communication techniques, non-pharmacological interventions, and medication, to manage the symptoms and improve the quality of life of individuals with dementia. However, it is important to tailor the approach to the individual's needs and preferences and to seek professional guidance when necessary.

Strategies for maintaining quality of life at each stage

Dementia is a progressive disease that affects different areas of the brain and can cause a range of symptoms. As the disease progresses, it can become more difficult for individuals to perform everyday tasks, maintain relationships, and communicate effectively. However, there are strategies that can help individuals with dementia maintain their quality of life and improve their overall well-being. These strategies may also benefit caregivers and family members who are supporting individuals with dementia.

In this section, we will discuss strategies for maintaining quality of life at each stage of dementia, including:

Early Stage Strategies

Middle Stage Strategies

Late Stage Strategies

Early Stage Strategies:

During the early stages of dementia, individuals may still be able to maintain their independence and participate in their usual activities. Some strategies that can help maintain quality of life during this stage include:

Staying active and engaged: Encourage individuals to continue participating in activities they enjoy, such as hobbies or exercise, as this can help them maintain their physical and mental well-being.

Promoting social interaction: Social interaction is important for maintaining cognitive function and overall well-being. Encourage individuals to spend time with friends and family, join social groups, or participate in community events.

Simplifying tasks: As dementia can make it difficult to perform complex tasks, simplify tasks and routines to help individuals maintain their independence and confidence.

Addressing safety concerns: Make necessary adaptations to the home environment to promote safety, such as removing tripping hazards or installing grab bars.

Middle Stage Strategies:

During the middle stages of dementia, individuals may require more assistance with daily tasks and experience more pronounced cognitive and physical symptoms. Strategies that can help maintain quality of life during this stage include:

Encouraging independence: While individuals may require assistance with some tasks, it's important to encourage independence and provide opportunities for individuals to participate in activities they enjoy.

Adapting the environment: Make adaptations to the home environment to help individuals maintain their independence, such as using visual cues to help with navigation or labeling drawers and cabinets.

Providing meaningful activities: Engage individuals in activities that are meaningful to them, such as listening to music, looking at photos, or participating in arts and crafts.

Addressing behavioral symptoms: Behavioral symptoms, such as agitation or aggression, may become more pronounced during the middle stages of dementia. Strategies such as distraction techniques, redirection, or relaxation techniques may be helpful.

Late Stage Strategies:

During the late stages of dementia, individuals may require more extensive care and support. Strategies that can help maintain quality of life during this stage include:

Providing comfort and support: Focus on providing comfort and support for the individual, such as through gentle touch or familiar music.

Addressing physical symptoms: As physical symptoms, such as difficulty swallowing or incontinence, may become more pronounced during the late stages of dementia, it's important to provide appropriate medical care and support.

Encouraging sensory stimulation: Engage the individual's senses, such as through music, aromatherapy, or soft textures, to promote comfort and relaxation.

Providing a supportive environment: Create a supportive environment that meets the individual's needs, such as through gentle lighting or familiar objects.

Overall, the strategies outlined above can help individuals with dementia maintain their quality of life and improve their overall well-being at each stage of the disease. Caregivers and family members can also benefit from these strategies, as they can help reduce stress and improve the caregiving experience.

Tips for caregivers and family members

Dementia is a complex and challenging disease, and caring for someone with dementia can be an emotional and stressful experience for family members and caregivers. Providing care for someone with dementia requires patience, empathy, and understanding, as well as knowledge of the disease and its progression. In this section, we will provide some tips and strategies for caregivers and family members to help manage the challenges of caring for someone with dementia.

Educate yourself about dementia

The first step in caring for someone with dementia is to educate yourself about the disease. Understanding the disease, its symptoms, and its progression can help you provide better care and support for your loved one. It's important to learn about the different types of dementia, the stages of the disease, and how it affects the brain and behavior. You can consult with healthcare professionals, attend support groups, and read books or articles about dementia to gain more knowledge and insights.

Create a routine

Creating a daily routine can help provide structure and stability for individuals with dementia, as well as for caregivers. Establishing a consistent routine for meals, activities, and rest can help individuals with dementia feel more secure and less anxious. It's important to be flexible and adapt the routine as needed, depending on the individual's needs and preferences.

Use effective communication strategies

Communicating with someone with dementia can be challenging, as the disease can affect their ability to understand and express themselves. Using effective communication strategies can help improve the quality of communication and reduce frustration for both the individual with dementia and the caregiver. Some effective communication strategies include speaking clearly and slowly, using simple language, providing visual cues, and listening actively.

Encourage physical and mental activities

Physical and mental activities can help improve the overall health and well-being of individuals with dementia. Engaging in physical activities such as walking, dancing, or gardening can help improve balance, mobility, and mood. Mental activities such as puzzles, games, or music can help stimulate the brain and provide a sense of accomplishment. It's important to find activities that the individual with dementia enjoys and is capable of doing.

Take care of yourself

Caring for someone with dementia can be emotionally and physically exhausting, and it's important for caregivers to take care of themselves as well. This can include getting enough rest, exercise, and nutrition, as well as seeking support from others. Caregivers can attend support groups, talk to friends or family members, or seek professional counseling to help manage stress and burnout.

Seek support and resources

Caring for someone with dementia can be overwhelming, and it's important for caregivers to seek support and resources. There are many resources available for caregivers, including support groups, respite care, and home health services. It's important to ask for help when needed and to build a network of support to help manage the challenges of caring for someone with dementia.

In conclusion, caring for someone with dementia can be challenging, but with the right knowledge, strategies, and support, caregivers and family members can provide effective care and improve the quality of life for individuals with dementia. By educating yourself about the disease, creating a routine, using effective communication strategies, encouraging physical and mental activities, taking care of yourself, and seeking support and resources, you can help manage the challenges of caring for someone with dementia and improve the overall well-being of your loved one.

Chapter 3: Approaches to Care and Treatment
Holistic approaches to care, including non-pharmacological interventions

Dementia is a complex condition that affects not only the cognitive abilities of the person with the disease but also their emotional, social, and physical well-being. Therefore, a holistic approach to care is essential for managing the symptoms and improving the quality of life for people with dementia. This chapter will explore non-pharmacological interventions and other holistic approaches to care that can be used to support people with dementia.

Non-pharmacological Interventions

Non-pharmacological interventions are approaches to care that do not involve medication. These interventions are often used as a first-line treatment for people with dementia because they have fewer side effects than medications and are generally safer. Non-pharmacological interventions include the following:

Cognitive Stimulation Therapy

Cognitive stimulation therapy involves a series of activities and exercises that are designed to improve cognitive function and promote social interaction. These activities may include word games, puzzles, and memory exercises. Cognitive stimulation therapy has been shown to improve cognitive function and quality of life for people with dementia.

Reminiscence Therapy

Reminiscence therapy involves recalling past experiences and events as a way of promoting social interaction and enhancing self-esteem. This therapy may involve looking at old photographs or listening to music from the person's past. Reminiscence therapy has been shown to improve mood and social interaction for people with dementia.

Validation Therapy

Validation therapy involves acknowledging the person's feelings and emotions and trying to understand their perspective. This therapy may involve using active listening techniques and asking open-ended questions to encourage the person to express themselves. Validation therapy has been shown to improve communication and reduce agitation for people with dementia.

Music Therapy

Music therapy involves using music to promote relaxation and improve mood. This therapy may involve listening to music or playing musical instruments. Music therapy has been shown to improve mood and reduce anxiety for people with dementia.

Pet Therapy

Pet therapy involves introducing animals into the person's environment as a way of promoting social interaction and reducing stress. This therapy may involve bringing in a trained therapy dog or cat. Pet therapy has been shown to reduce agitation and improve mood for people with dementia.

Other Holistic Approaches to Care

In addition to non-pharmacological interventions, there are other holistic approaches to care that can be used to support people with dementia. These approaches include the following:

Person-Centered Care

Person-centered care involves tailoring care to the individual needs and preferences of the person with dementia. This approach focuses on promoting independence, dignity, and respect for the person with dementia. Person-centered care has been shown to improve quality of life and reduce agitation for people with dementia.

Exercise

Exercise has been shown to improve physical health and cognitive function for people with dementia. Exercise may involve activities such as walking, swimming, or yoga.

Exercise has been shown to improve mood, reduce agitation, and improve sleep for people with dementia.

Nutrition

Good nutrition is essential for maintaining physical health and cognitive function for people with dementia. A healthy diet may include a variety of fruits, vegetables, whole grains, and lean protein. Good nutrition has been shown to improve physical health and cognitive function for people with dementia.

Sleep

Sleep is important for physical and cognitive health for people with dementia. Sleep hygiene may involve establishing a regular sleep routine, avoiding caffeine and alcohol before bedtime, and creating a comfortable sleep environment. Good sleep hygiene has been shown to improve cognitive function and reduce agitation for people with dementia.

Conclusion

Dementia is a complex condition that requires a holistic approach to care. Non-pharmacological interventions and other holistic approaches to care can be used to support people with dementia and improve their quality of life. Care should be tailored to meet the specific needs of each individual, taking into account their unique symptoms, personality, and preferences. Some non-pharmacological interventions that have been found to be effective in supporting people with dementia include music therapy, art therapy, reminiscence therapy, pet therapy, and aromatherapy. These interventions can help to reduce anxiety, agitation, and other challenging behaviors, as well as improve communication and social interaction. Additionally, exercise, healthy diet, and sleep hygiene can also be beneficial for people with dementia, helping to promote physical health and well-being, as well as cognitive function. Holistic care also involves providing emotional support and social engagement for individuals with dementia, helping them to maintain a sense of connection and purpose. This can involve engaging in meaningful activities, such as hobbies, socializing with friends and family, and participating in community events.

Medications and their potential benefits and side effects

Dementia is a progressive neurological disorder for which there is currently no cure. However, medications can be used to manage symptoms and slow down the progression of the disease. There are different types of medications used to treat dementia, and each has its own benefits and potential side effects. It is important to understand these medications to make informed decisions about their use.

Acetylcholinesterase inhibitors (AChEIs) are one type of medication commonly used to treat dementia. They work by increasing the levels of a neurotransmitter called acetylcholine in the brain, which is important for memory and learning. Three AChEIs are currently approved by the FDA for the treatment of Alzheimer's disease: donepezil (Aricept), rivastigmine (Exelon), and galantamine (Razadyne). These medications have been shown to improve cognitive function and activities of daily living, and to reduce behavioral symptoms in people with mild to moderate Alzheimer's disease. However, they do not work for everyone, and their benefits may be modest.

Another type of medication used to treat dementia is memantine (Namenda), an N-methyl-D-aspartate (NMDA) receptor antagonist. Memantine works by regulating glutamate, a neurotransmitter that is involved in learning and memory. It is approved for the treatment of moderate to severe Alzheimer's disease and can be used in combination with AChEIs. Studies have shown that memantine can improve cognitive function and activities of daily living, and may also reduce behavioral symptoms.

Antipsychotic medications may be prescribed to treat behavioral symptoms such as aggression, agitation, and hallucinations. However, these medications have significant side effects and should be used with caution. They are associated with an increased risk of stroke, falls, and mortality in people with dementia. It is recommended that they be used only for short-term treatment of severe behavioral symptoms and with close monitoring.

Other medications may be prescribed to treat specific symptoms, such as depression or sleep disturbances. It is important to discuss the potential benefits and risks of any medication with a healthcare provider before starting treatment. Medications may also interact with each other or with other health conditions, so it is important to provide a complete list of all medications and supplements being taken.

In addition to medications, there are other approaches to care and treatment that can be used to manage symptoms and improve quality of life for people with dementia. These include non-pharmacological interventions such as music therapy, pet therapy, and sensory stimulation, as well as lifestyle modifications such as exercise and a healthy diet. It is important to take a holistic approach to care and treatment, addressing not only the physical symptoms but also the emotional and social needs of the person with dementia and their caregivers.

Supportive services and resources for individuals with dementia and their caregivers

Individuals with dementia and their caregivers may benefit from accessing supportive services and resources that can help them navigate the challenges of living with this condition. There are various types of services and resources available that can provide assistance, education, and support for those affected by dementia.

One type of service that can be particularly helpful is respite care. Respite care provides temporary relief for caregivers by arranging for another person to take on caregiving responsibilities for a short period of time. This can be especially important for caregivers who may feel overwhelmed or burned out and need a break to recharge.

Another helpful resource for individuals with dementia and their caregivers is support groups. Support groups can provide a safe and supportive environment for individuals to share their experiences and connect with others who are going through similar situations. Support groups can be particularly beneficial for caregivers, who may feel isolated or misunderstood in their caregiving roles.

In addition to respite care and support groups, there are a variety of other supportive services and resources available for individuals with dementia and their caregivers. Some of these include:

Memory clinics: Memory clinics are specialized healthcare settings that provide comprehensive diagnostic evaluations, treatment, and ongoing management for individuals with dementia.

Home health care services: Home health care services can provide assistance with activities of daily living, medication management, and other healthcare needs in the home setting.

Elder law services: Elder law services can help individuals with dementia and their families navigate legal and financial issues related to caregiving, estate planning, and other related matters.

Technology-based resources: Technology-based resources, such as apps and devices designed specifically for individuals with dementia, can provide assistance with memory tasks, communication, and other needs.

It's important to note that accessing these services and resources may require navigating complex systems and funding sources, such as Medicaid or private insurance. However, many organizations and advocacy groups offer guidance and support for individuals and families seeking these types of services.

In addition to these formal services and resources, individuals with dementia and their caregivers may also benefit from informal support networks, such as friends, family members, and community groups. Building and maintaining these networks can help provide a sense of belonging, emotional support, and practical assistance to those affected by dementia.

In summary, there are a variety of supportive services and resources available for individuals with dementia and their caregivers. These resources can help improve quality of life, reduce stress, and provide much-needed assistance and support to those affected by this complex condition. It's important for individuals and families to explore these options and find the support that best meets their needs.

Legal and financial planning considerations for dementia patients and their families

Dementia is a progressive disease that not only affects a person's cognitive abilities but also their decision-making and financial planning abilities. As the disease progresses, individuals with dementia may have difficulty managing their finances and legal affairs, which can have significant consequences for both the patient and their family. Therefore, it is essential to plan ahead and make legal and financial arrangements while the person with dementia is still capable of making decisions.

Legal Planning:

Legal planning involves creating or updating legal documents to ensure that the person with dementia's wishes are respected and their affairs are managed appropriately. These legal documents may include a power of attorney (POA), living will, and guardianship. A POA is a legal document that grants another person the authority to make financial and legal decisions on behalf of the person with dementia. A living will is a legal document that specifies the person's medical treatment preferences if they become unable to communicate their wishes. Guardianship may be necessary when the person with dementia is no longer able to make decisions for themselves, and no POA is in place.

Financial Planning:

Financial planning involves managing the person's assets and income, including paying bills, managing investments, and ensuring that the person with dementia has adequate long-term care insurance. Financial planning also involves identifying potential scams and preventing financial exploitation of vulnerable individuals. Financial planning may include working with financial advisors, attorneys, and accountants to ensure that the person's finances are managed appropriately.

Resources and Support:

There are several resources and supportive services available for individuals with dementia and their families. Some of these resources include adult day care centers, respite care, in-home care, and support groups. Adult day care centers provide a safe and supportive environment for individuals with dementia to socialize and participate in activities, while respite care provides temporary relief to caregivers. In-home care may include personal care, such as assistance with bathing and dressing, and homemaking services, such as cleaning and meal preparation. Support groups provide emotional support and education to caregivers and family members.

Conclusion:

Legal and financial planning considerations for dementia patients and their families are essential to ensure that the person's wishes are respected, their assets are managed appropriately, and their affairs are in order. It is important to plan ahead and seek professional advice to ensure that the person's legal and financial needs are adequately addressed. Additionally, there are several resources and supportive services available to help individuals with dementia and their families navigate the challenges associated with the disease. By taking a proactive approach to legal and financial planning, individuals with dementia and their families can alleviate some of the stress and uncertainty associated with the disease.

Chapter 4: Creating a Supportive Environment
Adapting the home environment to promote safety and independence

As individuals with dementia progress through the different stages of the disease, their ability to perform daily activities may become compromised. As such, it is important to adapt the home environment to promote safety and independence. Some modifications may be simple, such as removing tripping hazards and ensuring adequate lighting. Other modifications may require more planning and may involve remodeling or renovation.

One important consideration when adapting the home environment is to ensure that it is easy to navigate. This may involve removing clutter and reorganizing furniture to create clear pathways. Additionally, it may be helpful to add visual cues, such as labels or pictures, to help individuals with dementia navigate their environment.

Another consideration when adapting the home environment is to make it easier for individuals with dementia to perform daily tasks. This may involve installing grab bars or handrails in the bathroom or kitchen, or providing specialized utensils to aid in eating.

When adapting the home environment, it is also important to consider the safety of the individual with dementia. This may involve installing locks on doors and windows, adding gates to stairways, and removing or locking up potentially dangerous items, such as sharp objects and cleaning supplies.

Finally, it is important to consider the emotional needs of the individual with dementia when adapting the home environment. Creating a warm and inviting space with familiar items, such as family photos and favorite books, can help individuals with dementia feel more comfortable and at ease in their surroundings. It may also be helpful to incorporate calming elements, such as soft lighting and soothing music.

Overall, adapting the home environment to promote safety and independence for individuals with dementia requires careful planning and consideration. By making modifications that address the specific needs of the individual with dementia, caregivers can create a supportive environment that promotes quality of life and enhances overall well-being.

Creating a social support network for individuals with dementia and their caregivers

Dementia can be a challenging condition for both the individual with dementia and their caregivers. Caregivers may feel overwhelmed, stressed, and isolated, and individuals with dementia may experience social isolation and loneliness. A social support network can help both the individual with dementia and their caregiver cope with the challenges of the condition and improve their quality of life. In this chapter, we will explore the importance of creating a social support network and provide tips on how to create one.

Importance of a social support network for individuals with dementia

Social support can take many forms, such as emotional support, informational support, and instrumental support. Emotional support involves providing empathy, love, and care, while informational support involves providing information and guidance. Instrumental support involves providing practical help, such as running errands, preparing meals, or assisting with transportation.

A social support network can provide all of these types of support, which can be crucial for individuals with dementia and their caregivers. A supportive network can provide emotional support and help both the individual with dementia and their caregiver feel less isolated and more connected to others. Informational support can be essential in helping caregivers navigate the complex healthcare system and understand the care and treatment options available. Instrumental support can help both the individual with dementia and their caregiver with day-to-day tasks and errands, reducing stress and improving quality of life.

Creating a social support network

Creating a social support network can be challenging, but it is essential for individuals with dementia and their caregivers. Here are some tips on how to create a supportive network:

Reach out to family and friends: Family and friends can be a great source of support. Reach out to them and let them know what you need. Ask for their help with specific tasks or simply spend time with them to reduce feelings of isolation.

Join a support group: Joining a support group can provide a sense of community and understanding. Support groups can be found through community centers, hospitals, and online resources.

Seek out professional support: Professional support can provide valuable resources and assistance. Seek out social workers, counselors, or other professionals who specialize in dementia care.

Consider respite care: Respite care can provide caregivers with a break from their caregiving duties. This can allow caregivers to take care of their own needs, reduce stress, and improve their ability to provide care.

Explore community resources: Community resources, such as adult day programs, transportation services, and meal delivery services, can be valuable resources for individuals with dementia and their caregivers.

Conclusion

Creating a social support network is essential for individuals with dementia and their caregivers. A supportive network can provide emotional, informational, and instrumental support, reducing feelings of isolation and stress and improving quality of life. Reach out to family and friends, join a support group, seek out professional support, consider respite care, and explore community resources to create a supportive network. By creating a social support network, individuals with dementia and their caregivers can feel less alone and better able to cope with the challenges of the condition.

Incorporating meaningful activities into daily life

Introduction: One of the key challenges for individuals with dementia is maintaining engagement in activities that bring purpose and joy to their lives. As dementia progresses, it can become increasingly difficult to engage in activities that were once enjoyed, leading to feelings of boredom and isolation. However, research has shown that incorporating meaningful activities into daily life can have numerous benefits for individuals with dementia, including improved mood, reduced agitation, and enhanced social connections. This section will explore the importance of meaningful activities for individuals with dementia and provide practical tips for incorporating such activities into daily life.

The Importance of Meaningful Activities for Individuals with Dementia: Engaging in meaningful activities can help individuals with dementia maintain their sense of self and identity, provide a sense of purpose, and promote feelings of accomplishment. Activities that were once enjoyed can also serve as a source of comfort and familiarity, helping to reduce anxiety and depression. Additionally, participating in activities with others can promote social connections and reduce feelings of isolation.

Tips for Incorporating Meaningful Activities into Daily Life:

Tailor activities to the individual's interests and abilities: When selecting activities, it is important to consider the individual's interests and abilities. Activities that were once enjoyed may need to be adapted as dementia progresses, but can still be meaningful with some modifications. For example, if an individual enjoyed gardening but is no longer able to perform physically demanding tasks, they could still participate in planting and caring for a small indoor garden.

Create a routine: Establishing a consistent routine can provide structure and predictability, reducing feelings of anxiety and confusion. Activities can be scheduled into the routine, such as a daily walk or an afternoon game of cards.

Provide opportunities for socialization: Social connections are important for individuals with dementia, and group activities can provide opportunities for socialization. Consider joining a support group or community center that offers activities tailored to individuals with dementia.

Use reminiscence therapy: Reminiscence therapy involves engaging in activities or conversations that evoke memories and stories from the individual's past. This can help promote feelings of connectedness and validation.

Incorporate sensory stimulation: Sensory stimulation activities can be engaging and enjoyable for individuals with dementia. Examples include listening to music, smelling flowers, or tactile activities such as sorting or folding laundry.

Offer choices: Offering choices can provide individuals with dementia with a sense of control and independence. For example, allowing the individual to choose between two activities or offering a choice in the time of day an activity is performed.

Conclusion: Incorporating meaningful activities into daily life can have numerous benefits for individuals with dementia. By tailoring activities to the individual's interests and abilities, creating a routine, providing opportunities for socialization, using reminiscence therapy, incorporating sensory stimulation, and offering choices, individuals with dementia can maintain a sense of purpose, reduce feelings of isolation, and improve their overall quality of life.

Addressing behavioral and psychological symptoms of dementia

Behavioral and psychological symptoms of dementia (BPSD) are common in people with dementia, and they can be challenging to manage. BPSD can include agitation, aggression, hallucinations, delusions, depression, anxiety, apathy, and sleep disturbances. These symptoms can be distressing for both the person with dementia and their caregivers. It is essential to address BPSD to improve the person's quality of life and prevent harm to themselves or others.

The causes of BPSD are complex and can be due to various factors, including pain, environmental triggers, medication side effects, and unmet needs. Therefore, a comprehensive approach that addresses the underlying causes is necessary for managing BPSD effectively.

Non-pharmacological interventions are the first-line approach for managing BPSD. These interventions are effective and have fewer side effects than pharmacological options. Non-pharmacological interventions focus on addressing the underlying causes of BPSD and promoting a supportive and safe environment for the person with dementia.

The following non-pharmacological interventions can be helpful in managing BPSD:

Validation therapy: Validation therapy involves acknowledging and accepting the person's feelings and emotions, even if they do not reflect reality. Validation therapy can reduce agitation, aggression, and anxiety in people with dementia.

Reminiscence therapy: Reminiscence therapy involves recalling positive memories and experiences from the person's past. Reminiscence therapy can improve mood, decrease agitation, and promote social interaction.

Music therapy: Music therapy involves listening to or singing songs, which can reduce agitation, improve mood, and increase social interaction.

Pet therapy: Pet therapy involves interacting with animals, such as dogs and cats, which can reduce agitation, anxiety, and depression and improve social interaction.

Multisensory stimulation: Multisensory stimulation involves stimulating the person's senses, such as touch, smell, and sight, with various objects and activities. Multisensory stimulation can reduce agitation, improve mood, and increase social interaction.

In some cases, pharmacological interventions may be necessary to manage BPSD. However, these medications should be used cautiously and only after non-pharmacological interventions have been tried. Antipsychotic medications can be effective in reducing agitation, aggression, and psychosis, but they have significant side effects and are associated with an increased risk of mortality in people with dementia. Therefore, the use of antipsychotic medications should be limited to severe cases and used under close supervision.

In conclusion, addressing BPSD is essential for improving the quality of life of people with dementia and their caregivers. Non-pharmacological interventions should be the first-line approach, and pharmacological interventions should be used with caution and under close supervision. A comprehensive approach that addresses the underlying causes of BPSD and promotes a supportive and safe environment is necessary for managing BPSD effectively.

Chapter 5: Addressing the Emotional Impact of Dementia

Coping with the emotional impact of a dementia diagnosis

Receiving a diagnosis of dementia can be an emotional and overwhelming experience for both the person with the condition and their loved ones. It can bring up a range of emotions, including fear, sadness, anger, and grief. Coping with these emotions can be a challenging process, but it is an important part of adjusting to life with dementia. Here are some strategies that may be helpful:

Educate yourself: Learning about dementia can help you and your loved ones better understand the condition and its effects. It can also help you feel more empowered and in control.

Seek support: Dementia can be isolating, but there are many sources of support available. This may include support groups, counseling, and online resources. Talking to others who are going through similar experiences can be a powerful source of comfort and validation.

Practice self-care: Caring for someone with dementia can be physically and emotionally taxing. It is important to prioritize self-care and take breaks when needed. This may include exercise, meditation, or engaging in hobbies that bring joy.

Address grief and loss: Dementia is a progressive condition, and it can be difficult to see a loved one's abilities decline over time. It is important to acknowledge and process feelings of grief and loss that may arise.

Focus on the present: Dwelling on the past or worrying about the future can be overwhelming. Focusing on the present moment and finding joy in small moments can help improve quality of life for both the person with dementia and their loved ones.

Communicate openly: Open and honest communication can help reduce stress and build stronger relationships. It is important to discuss concerns and feelings with loved ones and healthcare providers.

Find meaning and purpose: Living with dementia does not mean that life is over. Finding meaning and purpose can help bring a sense of fulfillment and joy to life. This may include participating in activities that align with personal values and beliefs, volunteering, or pursuing creative outlets.

In summary, receiving a diagnosis of dementia can be a difficult and emotional experience. Coping with these emotions is an important part of adjusting to life with the condition. By seeking support, practicing self-care, addressing grief and loss, focusing on the present, communicating openly, and finding meaning and purpose, it is possible to find joy and fulfillment in life with dementia.

Managing stress and burnout as a caregiver

Caring for a loved one with dementia can be a rewarding experience, but it can also be stressful and emotionally challenging. Caregivers may experience a range of emotions, including sadness, frustration, guilt, and anger. Over time, these emotions can build up and lead to burnout, a state of physical, emotional, and mental exhaustion. Burnout can cause caregivers to feel overwhelmed, exhausted, and unable to cope with their responsibilities.

To avoid burnout and manage stress, caregivers need to prioritize their own physical and emotional well-being. Here are some strategies that can help:

Seek support: Caregivers need to know that they are not alone. Joining a support group or talking to a trusted friend or family member can help caregivers feel understood and supported. Online support groups and forums can also be a helpful resource.

Take breaks: Caregivers need to take regular breaks to recharge and engage in self-care. This can include taking a walk, reading a book, or practicing meditation. Even short breaks can help caregivers feel more refreshed and energized.

Set boundaries: Caregivers need to set realistic boundaries around their caregiving responsibilities. This may mean delegating tasks to other family members or hiring a professional caregiver to provide respite care.

Practice self-care: Caregivers need to prioritize their own physical and emotional health. This can include getting enough sleep, eating a healthy diet, and engaging in regular exercise. Caregivers also need to engage in activities that bring them joy and fulfillment, such as hobbies or spending time with friends.

Seek professional help: Caregivers may benefit from counseling or therapy to help them manage their emotions and cope with the challenges of caregiving. Professional help can also be beneficial for addressing any mental health issues that may arise as a result of caregiving.

Learn to recognize and manage stress: Caregivers need to learn to recognize the signs of stress and implement strategies to manage it. This may include deep breathing exercises, visualization, or progressive muscle relaxation.

Practice gratitude: Caregivers can benefit from practicing gratitude and focusing on the positive aspects of their caregiving experience. This can help them feel more resilient and better able to cope with the challenges of caregiving.

In addition to these strategies, caregivers need to remember that it is okay to ask for help and take time for themselves. By prioritizing their own well-being, caregivers can provide better care for their loved ones with dementia and avoid burnout.

Support and resources for family members and caregivers

Caring for someone with dementia can be a challenging and emotional experience for family members and caregivers. It is essential to recognize the importance of self-care and the availability of support and resources to help alleviate some of the stress and burden that caregivers may experience. In this section, we will discuss some of the support and resources available to family members and caregivers of individuals with dementia.

Support groups: Support groups provide a safe and confidential space for family members and caregivers to share their experiences, emotions, and concerns. These groups offer emotional support, practical advice, and an opportunity to connect with others who are going through similar experiences. Support groups can be in-person or online, and there are many options available, including general caregiver support groups, dementia-specific groups, and groups that cater to specific cultural or language needs.

Respite care: Respite care provides temporary relief for caregivers by arranging for someone else to care for their loved one with dementia for a short period. This break can be essential for caregivers' mental and physical well-being, allowing them to rest, recharge, and take care of other responsibilities. Respite care can be provided in-home or at a care facility, and there are many options available depending on the needs and preferences of the family.

Home care services: Home care services offer support and assistance to individuals with dementia in their homes. These services can include personal care, such as bathing and dressing, housekeeping, meal preparation, medication reminders, and companionship. Home care services can be arranged through an agency or privately hired, and there are different levels of care available, depending on the individual's needs.

Adult day programs: Adult day programs provide a structured and safe environment for individuals with dementia to participate in meaningful activities and socialize with others while giving caregivers a break. These programs can also provide health monitoring, medication management, and personal care services. Adult day programs can be beneficial for both the individual with dementia and the caregiver, providing socialization and stimulation for the individual and relief and respite for the caregiver.

Educational resources: Educational resources can help family members and caregivers better understand dementia and how to manage it. There are many resources available, including books, websites, online courses, and workshops. These resources can provide information on the different stages of dementia, strategies for managing symptoms, communication techniques, and tips for self-care and stress management.

Professional counseling: Professional counseling can provide emotional support and guidance to family members and caregivers dealing with the challenges of caring for someone with dementia. Counseling can help caregivers process their emotions, develop coping strategies, and improve their communication skills. Counseling can be provided by a licensed therapist or counselor and can be done in-person or online.

Financial and legal resources: Caring for someone with dementia can be costly, and there may be legal considerations to take into account, such as power of attorney and advanced directives. There are many resources available to help navigate these issues, including financial advisors, elder law attorneys, and government assistance programs. It is essential to plan for the future and address these issues early on to alleviate some of the stress and burden on the caregiver.

In conclusion, caring for someone with dementia can be emotionally and physically exhausting, but it is essential to recognize the importance of self-care and the availability of support and resources to help alleviate some of the burden. Family members and caregivers can benefit from support groups, respite care, home care services, adult day programs, educational resources, professional counseling, and financial and legal resources. It is crucial to take advantage of these resources to ensure the best possible quality of life for both the individual with dementia and their caregiver.

Finding joy and connection in the midst of dementia

Caring for someone with dementia can be a challenging and emotional journey. As a caregiver, it can be easy to become consumed with the daily demands and the overwhelming nature of the disease. However, it is important to remember that there are still moments of joy and connection that can be found throughout the journey. In this section, we will explore ways to find joy and connection in the midst of dementia, and how to incorporate these moments into your daily routine.

Maintaining a Sense of Connection:

One of the most important ways to find joy in the midst of dementia is to maintain a sense of connection with the person you are caring for. This can be done through a variety of activities and gestures, such as:

Engaging in familiar activities: Try to engage in activities that the person with dementia enjoys and finds comforting. This could be listening to music, reading a book, or doing a puzzle together. Even simple activities like taking a walk or sitting outside in the sun can be a source of joy and connection.

Expressing love and affection: Even though the person with dementia may not always remember who you are, expressing your love and affection can still have a positive impact on their well-being. Simple gestures like holding their hand or giving them a hug can help them feel loved and connected.

Sharing memories: Sharing memories of the person's past can be a powerful way to connect with them and bring joy to their day. This could be looking at old photo albums or reminiscing about a special event or moment in their life.

Creating a sensory-rich environment: Engage the senses with things like music, familiar smells, or favorite foods. These sensory experiences can evoke memories and emotions that can help the person feel more connected to their surroundings and the people around them.

Finding Joy in Everyday Moments:

In addition to maintaining a sense of connection, it is also important to look for joy in everyday moments. This can include:

Celebrating small victories: Whether it's a good day or simply a good moment, take time to celebrate the positive moments that happen throughout the day. This could be something as simple as a smile or a kind word.

Embracing humor: Laughter can be a powerful tool for reducing stress and bringing joy to the caregiving experience. Look for moments of humor in everyday situations and try to find ways to incorporate laughter into your daily routine.

Engaging in self-care: As a caregiver, it is important to prioritize your own well-being. Make time for activities that bring you joy, whether it's exercise, reading a book, or spending time with friends. Taking care of yourself will help you be better equipped to find joy in the caregiving experience.

Conclusion:

Caring for someone with dementia can be a challenging and emotional journey, but it is important to remember that there are still moments of joy and connection that can be found throughout the experience. By maintaining a sense of connection, finding joy in everyday moments, and prioritizing self-care, caregivers can help themselves and the person they are caring for find joy and connection in the midst of dementia.

Chapter 6: Living with Dementia: Insights from Personal Experiences

Real-life stories of individuals and families living with dementia

Dementia affects millions of individuals and their families around the world. Each person's experience with dementia is unique, but sharing personal stories and insights can help to reduce the isolation and stigma that often surrounds the condition. In this chapter, we will explore real-life stories of individuals and families living with dementia, highlighting the challenges they face and the strategies they use to cope.

Mary's Story

Mary was diagnosed with early-onset Alzheimer's disease in her early sixties. Her husband, John, became her primary caregiver, but he struggled to balance his job and caregiving responsibilities. Mary's condition worsened, and she eventually moved into a memory care facility. John continued to visit her daily and found comfort in spending time with other caregivers who understood what he was going through.

Carlos's Story

Carlos was diagnosed with Lewy body dementia in his late seventies. His wife, Maria, became his caregiver, but she was not familiar with the condition and found it challenging to manage his symptoms. Carlos experienced hallucinations and often became agitated. Maria reached out to a local support group for caregivers of individuals with dementia and found a community of people who provided emotional support and practical advice.

Sarah's Story

Sarah's mother, Rachel, was diagnosed with dementia when Sarah was in her twenties. As Rachel's condition progressed, Sarah became her primary caregiver. She struggled with the emotional toll of caregiving and felt guilty for feeling resentful at times. Sarah sought therapy and found a support group for young caregivers, which helped her to develop coping strategies and connect with others who were going through similar experiences.

William's Story

William was diagnosed with vascular dementia in his late seventies. His wife, Margaret, became his caregiver and struggled with the loss of their shared identity as a couple. She felt like her role had become solely that of a caregiver, and she missed their previous activities and social life. Margaret reached out to a local organization that offered respite care for individuals with dementia, which allowed her to take breaks and participate in activities that she enjoyed.

Jennifer's Story

Jennifer's father, David, was diagnosed with dementia when she was in her thirties. She struggled with the decision to move him into a memory care facility but ultimately realized that it was the best option for his safety and well-being. Jennifer visited him regularly and found comfort in connecting with other family members of residents.

Michael's Story

Michael's mother, Joan, was diagnosed with Alzheimer's disease when he was in his forties. He struggled with the emotional impact of watching her decline and felt overwhelmed by the caregiving responsibilities. Michael sought therapy and joined a support group for male caregivers, which helped him to develop coping strategies and connect with other men who were going through similar experiences.

These stories highlight the diverse experiences of individuals and families living with dementia. While the challenges of dementia can be overwhelming, finding community, support, and coping strategies can help to improve quality of life for both individuals with dementia and their caregivers. It's important to remember that seeking help is not a sign of weakness and that support is available for those who need it.

Challenges faced and lessons learned

Dementia is a challenging condition that can bring about a wide range of physical, emotional, and cognitive changes that can affect the individual and their loved ones. People living with dementia and their families face numerous challenges and must navigate the complexities of the condition on a daily basis. In this section, we will explore some of the challenges faced by individuals and families living with dementia, as well as the lessons that can be learned from their experiences.

One of the most significant challenges faced by individuals with dementia is the loss of independence. As the condition progresses, the individual may have difficulty performing even the most basic activities of daily living, such as bathing, dressing, and eating. This can be particularly challenging for family members, who may feel helpless or overwhelmed by the responsibility of providing care. Additionally, the changes in the person's personality and behavior can make communication difficult, leading to frustration and tension between the individual with dementia and their loved ones.

Another challenge faced by individuals with dementia and their families is the stigma associated with the condition. Dementia is often misunderstood, and individuals living with the condition may face discrimination or isolation from their communities. This can further exacerbate feelings of loneliness and isolation, which can be particularly difficult for individuals with dementia and their caregivers.

Despite these challenges, many families find ways to cope with and adapt to the changes brought about by dementia. By working together, they are able to find joy and meaning in their lives, even in the midst of the difficulties.

One common theme that emerges from the experiences of individuals and families living with dementia is the importance of staying connected to others. Whether it is through participating in social activities or connecting with support groups, staying connected can help to combat the isolation and loneliness that often accompany the condition.

Another lesson that can be learned from these experiences is the importance of planning ahead. This includes not only financial and legal planning, but also planning for the individual's care and support needs as the condition progresses. By planning ahead, families can ensure that their loved one's needs are met and that they receive the best possible care.

Additionally, many families emphasize the importance of finding joy and meaning in everyday activities. This can include engaging in hobbies or other activities that the individual enjoys, as well as focusing on the positive aspects of life and cherishing moments of connection with loved ones.

In conclusion, living with dementia can be challenging, but by working together and finding ways to adapt, individuals and families can learn valuable lessons and find joy and meaning in their lives. By sharing their experiences and insights, they can help others facing similar challenges and contribute to a greater understanding of the condition.

Coping strategies and tips for living well with dementia

A diagnosis of dementia can be overwhelming and life-changing for both the person with dementia and their loved ones. However, there are various coping strategies and tips that can help individuals with dementia and their families live well and maintain a good quality of life. Here are some practical tips:

Stay organized: Dementia can affect a person's memory and ability to plan and organize daily activities. Creating a daily routine and using reminders, such as a calendar or a whiteboard, can help the person with dementia stay on track and reduce anxiety.

Engage in physical activity: Regular physical activity can improve physical and mental health and reduce the risk of other health problems. Gentle exercises such as walking, yoga, or swimming can be enjoyable and beneficial for people with dementia.

Stay socially active: Social connections are essential for maintaining a good quality of life. Activities such as joining a support group or attending social events can help the person with dementia feel connected to others and reduce feelings of isolation.

Maintain a healthy diet: Eating a healthy and balanced diet can improve overall health and reduce the risk of other health problems. Including plenty of fruits, vegetables, whole grains, and lean protein can provide essential nutrients and energy.

Manage stress: Stress can worsen symptoms of dementia and affect overall well-being. Engaging in relaxation techniques such as deep breathing or meditation can help reduce stress and promote a sense of calm.

Stay mentally active: Engaging in mentally stimulating activities such as puzzles, reading, or playing games can help maintain cognitive function and delay the progression of dementia.

Seek support: Seeking support from healthcare professionals, support groups, or family and friends can provide emotional support and practical advice for managing the challenges of living with dementia.

In addition to these coping strategies, it's important to remember that every person with dementia is unique and may require different strategies for managing their symptoms and maintaining a good quality of life. Regular communication with healthcare professionals and loved ones can help ensure that the person with dementia receives individualized care and support. It's also important to be patient and understanding, as dementia can affect a person's behavior and communication. With the right support and care, it's possible for individuals with dementia to continue living fulfilling lives.

Inspiring stories of resilience and hope

Dementia can be a challenging and often heartbreaking condition to live with, both for the individuals diagnosed with it and their families and caregivers. However, amidst the difficulties and struggles, there are also inspiring stories of resilience, hope, and positivity that can provide comfort and encouragement to those affected by the disease.

These stories come from people living with dementia, their families, and caregivers who have found ways to live well and maintain a sense of purpose, joy, and connection despite the challenges.

One such story is that of Kate Swaffer, an Australian woman who was diagnosed with early-onset dementia at the age of 49. Instead of giving up, Kate became an advocate for people with dementia and a champion for their rights. She started a blog, authored several books, and founded the Dementia Alliance International, a global organization run by people with dementia. Kate's inspiring journey shows that a dementia diagnosis does not have to define or limit a person's life.

Another inspiring story is that of Norman McNamara, who was diagnosed with dementia at the age of 50. Norman refused to let his diagnosis define him, and instead, he decided to use his experience to raise awareness and funds for dementia research. He started the Purple Angel Dementia Campaign, which aims to improve dementia care and support worldwide. Norman's determination and passion for making a difference in the lives of people with dementia are truly inspiring.

There are also numerous examples of families and caregivers who have found ways to support their loved ones with dementia while maintaining their own well-being. For example, some families have created memory boxes or collages filled with meaningful objects or photographs that spark memories and provide comfort to their loved ones with dementia. Others have incorporated music, art, or other activities into their daily routines, providing opportunities for joy and connection.

These inspiring stories remind us that dementia does not have to be a death sentence or a life devoid of meaning and purpose. With the right support, resources, and mindset, people with dementia and their families can continue to live fulfilling and meaningful lives.

Conclusion

Recap of key takeaways from the book

In conclusion, this book has covered a wide range of topics related to dementia, including its causes, symptoms, diagnosis, and treatment options. It has also addressed the emotional impact of dementia on both the individual with dementia and their caregivers, as well as strategies for coping and finding joy in the midst of this challenging journey.

Throughout the book, several key takeaways have emerged that are worth highlighting in this final chapter. Firstly, it is important to recognize that dementia is a complex condition that affects individuals in unique ways. While there are common symptoms and behaviors associated with dementia, each person's experience is different, and therefore requires individualized care and support.

Secondly, a holistic approach to care is essential in supporting individuals with dementia. This approach should encompass not only medical treatment but also non-pharmacological interventions, supportive services, and a well-adapted home environment. By taking a holistic approach, individuals with dementia can maintain their independence and quality of life for as long as possible.

Thirdly, caregiving for someone with dementia can be both rewarding and challenging. It is important for caregivers to take care of themselves and seek support when needed to prevent burnout and maintain their own well-being.

Fourthly, individuals with dementia and their caregivers can benefit from a strong support network, including family, friends, and community resources. Support groups, counseling, and respite care can all provide valuable emotional and practical support.

Finally, it is important to remember that individuals with dementia can still lead meaningful and fulfilling lives. While the condition can bring significant challenges, there are also opportunities for joy, connection, and personal growth.

In summary, this book has provided a comprehensive overview of dementia and the various aspects involved in supporting individuals with the condition. By taking a holistic approach to care, seeking support, and finding joy in the journey, individuals with dementia and their caregivers can navigate this challenging experience with resilience and hope.

Call to action for readers to engage with and support the elder population living with dementia in their communities

As we conclude this book, it is important to reflect on the key takeaways we have explored in the previous chapters. We have learned about the different types of dementia, the risk factors, and warning signs to look out for. We have also explored the various approaches to care and treatment, including medications, supportive services, adapting the home environment, and addressing the emotional impact of dementia. Moreover, we have heard inspiring stories of resilience and hope from individuals and families living with dementia.

One of the most critical takeaways from this book is the importance of a holistic approach to dementia care. It is crucial to recognize that dementia affects not only the individual with the diagnosis but also their families and caregivers. We must ensure that they receive adequate support and resources to cope with the emotional, physical, and financial challenges that come with caring for someone with dementia.

We have also learned that meaningful connections and engagement in activities can significantly improve the quality of life for individuals with dementia. Caregivers and loved ones can play a crucial role in helping people with dementia find purpose and joy in their daily lives.

However, it is not enough to address dementia care on an individual or family level alone. As a society, we must recognize the growing population of older adults and the increasing prevalence of dementia. It is our responsibility to engage with and support the elder population living with dementia in our communities.

We can start by advocating for policies that prioritize dementia care and funding research that will lead to better treatments and potential cures. We can also volunteer our time and resources to support local organizations that provide services and resources for individuals and families affected by dementia.

In conclusion, the insights and knowledge gained from this book can help us navigate the complex world of dementia care. However, it is up to us to take action and support those affected by this debilitating condition. We must work together to create a world where individuals with dementia can live with dignity, purpose, and joy.

Final thoughts and encouragement for readers to navigate the complexities of dementia with empathy, understanding, and resilience

Dementia can be a challenging and complex condition that affects not only the individuals living with it but also their families and caregivers. While there is no cure for dementia, there are many ways to provide support, care, and resources to those affected by it. As we come to the end of this book, it is important to reflect on what we have learned and to encourage readers to approach dementia with empathy, understanding, and resilience.

Recap of Key Takeaways from the Book:

Throughout this book, we have covered various topics related to dementia, including its symptoms, diagnosis, treatment, and care. We have also explored the emotional impact of dementia on individuals and families, as well as strategies for coping and finding joy amidst the challenges.

Some of the key takeaways from this book include:

Dementia is not a normal part of aging but a neurological disorder that affects memory, cognition, and behavior.

Early diagnosis and treatment can help improve quality of life and delay the progression of symptoms.

Medications can be effective in managing some of the symptoms of dementia, but they also have potential side effects.

Creating a supportive environment that promotes safety, independence, and social connections can help individuals with dementia thrive.

Caregiving for someone with dementia can be emotionally and physically demanding, and it is important to seek support and resources.

Finding joy and meaning in everyday activities, connecting with others, and embracing humor and creativity can enhance quality of life for individuals with dementia and their families.

Call to Action:

As the population ages, the number of individuals living with dementia is expected to rise, and it is important that we all do our part to support this vulnerable population. Whether you are a family member, friend, neighbor, or community member, there are many ways you can engage with and support individuals with dementia and their families.

Here are some ways to get involved:

Educate yourself about dementia and its impact on individuals and families. Share what you learn with others to raise awareness and reduce stigma.

Volunteer with organizations that support individuals with dementia and their families, such as local Alzheimer's Association chapters or memory care facilities.

Offer to help families affected by dementia with tasks such as grocery shopping, meal preparation, or transportation.

Join or start a support group for caregivers of individuals with dementia. This can be a valuable source of emotional support and practical advice.

Advocate for policies that support individuals with dementia and their families, such as increased funding for research, caregiver support programs, and dementia-friendly communities.

Final Thoughts:

Living with dementia can be a difficult and emotional journey, but it is important to remember that individuals with dementia can still find joy, meaning, and connection in their lives. By approaching dementia with empathy, understanding, and resilience, we can help support individuals with dementia and their families in living their best lives.

As we close this book, I encourage readers to continue learning, engaging, and advocating for the elder population living with dementia in our communities. Together, we can make a positive difference in the lives of those affected by this complex condition.

THE END

Key Terms and Definitions

Key Terms and Definitions

To help you better understand the language and concepts related to aging and older adults, below you will find a list of key terms and their definitions.

Dementia: A decline in cognitive function that interferes with daily activities, characterized by memory loss, impaired communication, and difficulty with reasoning and problem-solving.

Alzheimer's disease: A progressive brain disorder that causes memory loss, impaired thinking, and behavioral changes.

Mild cognitive impairment: A mild decline in cognitive function that is greater than expected for age and education but does not interfere significantly with daily activities.

Neurodegeneration: The gradual loss of nerve cells in the brain, leading to a decline in cognitive function.

Caregiver: A person who provides physical, emotional, or financial support to an individual with dementia.

Activities of Daily Living (ADLs): Basic self-care tasks, such as bathing, dressing, and eating, that are necessary for independent living.

Instrumental Activities of Daily Living (IADLs): Complex tasks, such as managing finances, preparing meals, and driving, that are necessary for independent living.

Sundowning: A phenomenon in which individuals with dementia become more agitated and confused in the late afternoon or evening.

Wandering: A common behavior in which individuals with dementia wander aimlessly and may become lost or disoriented.

Respite care: Temporary care provided to relieve a primary caregiver of their responsibilities and provide a break from caregiving duties.

Palliative care: Specialized medical care focused on providing relief from symptoms and improving quality of life for individuals with serious illnesses, including dementia.

Advance directive: Legal document that specifies an individual's wishes regarding medical treatment and end-of-life care in the event they are unable to make decisions for themselves.

Power of attorney: Legal document that grants an individual the authority to make legal and financial decisions on behalf of another person.

Hospice care: Specialized care focused on providing comfort and support to individuals with terminal illnesses, including dementia, and their families.

Person-centered care: Approach to caregiving that focuses on the unique needs and preferences of the individual with dementia, emphasizing their dignity, autonomy, and quality of life.

Supporting Materials

Introduction:

Alzheimer's Association. (2021). 2021 Alzheimer's disease facts and figures. Alzheimer's & Dementia, 17(3), 327-406.

World Health Organization. (2017). Global action plan on the public health response to dementia 2017-2025. WHO Press.

Chapter 1: Understanding Dementia:

Alzheimer's Association. (2021). What is dementia? https://www.alz.org/alzheimers-dementia/what-is-dementia

Mayo Clinic. (2021). Dementia. https://www.mayoclinic.org/diseases-conditions/dementia/symptoms-causes/syc-20352013

National Institute on Aging. (2021). What is dementia? https://www.nia.nih.gov/health/what-dementia-symptoms-types-and-diagnosis

Chapter 2: Navigating Symptoms and Progression:

American Psychiatric Association. (2013). Diagnostic and statistical manual of mental disorders (5th ed.). American Psychiatric Publishing.

McKeith, I. G., Boeve, B. F., Dickson, D. W., et al. (2017). Diagnosis and management of dementia with Lewy bodies:

Fourth consensus report of the DLB Consortium. Neurology, 89(1), 88-100.

National Institute on Aging. (2021). Understanding Alzheimer's disease: Symptoms and stages. https://www.nia.nih.gov/health/understanding-alzheimers-disease-symptoms-stages

Chapter 3: Approaches to Care and Treatment:

Alzheimer's Association. (2021). Treatment and care. https://www.alz.org/alzheimers-dementia/treatments

National Institute on Aging. (2021). Alzheimer's and dementia care: Caregiving for the person with dementia. https://www.nia.nih.gov/health/alzheimers-and-dementia-caregiving/person-dementia

Chapter 4: Creating a Supportive Environment:

Alzheimer's Association. (2021). Home safety for people with Alzheimer's or dementia. https://www.alz.org/help-support/caregiving/safety/home-safety

National Institute on Aging. (2021). Home safety for people with Alzheimer's disease. https://www.nia.nih.gov/health/home-safety-people-alzheimers-disease

World Health Organization. (2019). Risk reduction of cognitive decline and dementia: WHO guidelines. WHO Press.

Chapter 5: Addressing the Emotional Impact of Dementia:

Alzheimer's Association. (2021). Coping with caregiving: The emotional journey. https://www.alz.org/help-support/caregiving/coping-with-caregiving/emotional-impact

National Institute on Aging. (2021). Alzheimer's caregiving: Coping with emotions. https://www.nia.nih.gov/health/alzheimers-caregiving-coping-emotions

Sherman, C. W., & Burgio, L. D. (2016). Coping with caregiver burnout and dementia-related behavioral issues. Journal of Gerontological Nursing, 42(2), 38-46.

Chapter 6: Living with Dementia: Insights from Personal Experiences:

Alzheimer's Association. (2021). Living with Alzheimer's and dementia: Personal stories. https://www.alz.org/stories

Nakanishi, M., & Nakashima, T. (2014). Living with dementia: A meta-synthesis of qualitative research on the lived experience. Geriatric Nursing, 35(5), 397-403.

Conclusion

Alzheimer's Association. (2021). 2021 Alzheimer's Disease Facts and Figures. https://www.alz.org/media/Documents/alzheimers-facts-and-figures.pdf

Brodaty, H., & Donkin, M. (2009). Family caregivers of people with dementia. Dialogues in clinical neuroscience, 11(2), 217-228.

Department of Health and Human Services. (2017). National Plan to Address Alzheimer's Disease. https://aspe.hhs.gov/pdf-report/national-plan-address-alzheimers-disease-2017-update

National Institute on Aging. (2021). Alzheimer's Disease and Related Dementias Research Milestones. https://www.nia.nih.gov/research/milestones

Prince, M., Wimo, A., Guerchet, M., Ali, G. C., Wu, Y. T., & Prina, M. (2015). World Alzheimer Report 2015: The Global Impact of Dementia. Alzheimer's Disease International.

Robinson, L., & Clare, L. (2011). Awareness in dementia: a review of assessment methods and measures. Aging & Mental Health, 15(8), 971-1040.

World Health Organization. (2017). Global action plan on the public health response to dementia 2017-2025. https://apps.who.int/iris/bitstream/handle/10665/259615/9789241513487-eng.pdf;jsessionid=FF35A325DAB7EFE38163B9E88A3D3B3A?sequence=1

Yates, L. A., & Leung, P. (2019). Enhancing person-centred care for people with dementia. British Journal of Nursing, 28(5), 302-306.

www.ingramcontent.com/pod-product-compliance
Lightning Source LLC
LaVergne TN
LVHW012122070526
838202LV00056B/5828